IIFYM Flexible Dieting

Sculpt The Perfect Body While Eating The Foods You Love

By Susan T. Williams

This book is designed to provide information on the topic covered. The information herein is offered for informational purposes solely. It is sold with the understanding that neither the author nor the publisher is engaged in rendering legal, accounting or other professional services. If legal or other professional advice is warranted, the services of an appropriate professional should be sought.

While every effort has been made to make the information presented here as complete and accurate as possible, it may contain errors, omissions or information that was accurate as of its publication but subsequently has become outdated by marketplace or industry changes. Neither author nor publisher accepts any liability or responsibility to any person or entity with respect to any loss or damage alleged to have been caused, directly or indirectly, by the information, ideas, opinions or other content in this book.

In no way, is it legal to reproduce, duplicate, or transmit any part of this document in either electronic means or printed form. Recording of this publication is strictly prohibited and any storage of this document is not allowed unless with written permission from the publisher.

The use of any trademark within this book is for clarifying purposes only, and any trademarks referenced in this work are used are without consent, and remain the property of the respective trademark holders, who are not affiliated with the publisher or this book.

Table of Contents

Introduction

Are you ready for a change? Are you tired of waking up in the morning and dreading the day that is waiting for you? Is your weight a constant problem? Are you tired of starting a new program every few weeks only to find that you have to quit because the program conflicts with your lifestyle too much? Or are you a hardcore athlete that is looking for the next step in your progression, yet you continually hit plateaus in your training? Do you want this to be the summer you put on that bathing suit you've been dreaming of for years?

The bad news is that it's all up to you.
But... the good news is, it's all up to you!

This book is written with YOU in mind. The programs are flexible, the food choices provide many, many options, and the schedule is designed by you. Everything that takes place from this point forward is designed to help you! It doesn't matter where you are in your life, this program can help you make your life better. You can wake up in the morning and feel excited about the possibilities in front of you. You can eliminate the pain you feel when you get out of bed and strengthen joints and muscles that have been dormant for too long. The serious competitor can take their workouts to a whole new level and accomplish a new set of goals. The IIFYM diet and wellness plan is for anyone, at any age, at any fitness level. All that remains is for you to make a decision to change your life, one small step at a time.

This book provides a detailed explanation of the If It Fits Your Macros diet, as well as offering a specific workout plan and a plethora of taste-tested recipes to assist you on your journey towards better health and wellness. As you read through this book, start to imagine how you can take the meals that you eat every day and fit them into this plan in one form or another. You may need to adjust some things like sauces, the method of cooking, the form of a protein or carbohydrate, or the amount consumed, but there is more than likely a way to incorporate many of your current favorites into this plan.

With the way our daily lives run us all ragged, having flexibility in a diet plan is absolutely necessary. Those rigid, structured plans that don't allow for cheat days and don't offer any forgiveness when we inevitably give-in are quickly becoming things of the past. The modern world is fast moving, and we have to stay as healthy as we possibly can if we are going to try to keep up with it. This book will show you how to do just that.

If you are ready to try something new, or even try a new way of looking at the same old foods and lifestyle choices, then this book will help you tremendously. Are you ready to take that first step? Can you make that leap of faith and really go for it? You can, if you simply take things one step at a time. Get on board and come along for the ride. You are not alone in your quest for a new way of eating and living. I know that you will find what you are looking for.

CHAPTER 1

The Plan

For the individual looking to improve their health, lose weight or gain self-confidence, there are plenty of popular diet plans to choose from. Each plan comes with its own promises and its own rules to follow. Some simply issue broad-based directives, such as cutting carbs or counting calories, and then fade off into the darkness when you start to search for specific instructions and guidelines to help you succeed over the long term. These diets present a one size fits all plan to the masses, and then the individual is supposed to find a way to tailor that plan to their needs.

This book provides a way for you to avoid those empty promises that lead to hopes being dashed. This book presents a detailed path for the reader to follow that is specifically programmed to their particular body type and goals. As you read through the examples, take a moment and fill in your own information on a piece of paper. Work through the formulas as you read along. This will allow you to literally custom design your own program as you progress through the chapters. It may be a little scary at first, and you may stumble a few times. If you do, just dust yourself off and take another step. You're not alone.

The IIFYM diet is a flexible method for eating a variety of foods while still keeping yourself on track to reach your goals. Unlike other diet plans that explicitly forbid fats, carbs, junk food, cheat days and the like, this plan allows for any number of flexible options, as long as those options fit into your prescribed calorie limit, fat content, protein quota and carbohydrate limit. As you examine the formula, begin to imagine how your own favorite foods may be able to fit into different segments of this program. You will be surprised by how easily you can adapt what you are currently eating to the program.

The IIFYM diet focuses on four main components: total calories, total protein, total carbs and total fat. This diet relies on measuring those "macro" nutrients we have just named in both grams and calories. In order to keep our measurements consistent, go ahead and write down the following rules:

1 gram of protein = 4 calories
1 gram of carbohydrates = 4 calories
1 gram of fat = 9 calories

These rules are the foundation for figuring the amount of macro nutrients you must consume and in what proportions. These rules never change and are held as a constant in the upcoming calculations.

Now that you know how many calories are in a gram, you are probably wondering how many grams of each nutrient you will need. This is where the individualization of the program begins. In order to set up your daily dietary goals, you must know your current weight, and you must decide on a target weight to use as your goal. The IIFYM diet is set up so that the user will need to consume the following amounts of macro nutrients, as it relates to their *desired* weight.

For proteins, the consumption is the same whether your goal is to gain or lose weight. Protein builds muscle and strengthens ligaments. Therefore, you will consume the following:

1 gram of protein for each pound of your desired body weight.

For carbohydrates, the consumption drastically changes depending on whether your goal is to lose weight or to gain weight. The exact amounts are directly related to the goal. If the goal is to lose weight, the prescibed amount decreases. If the goal is to gain weight, then the consumption increases. Here is a good guideline to use:

Fat Loss: Consume 1 gram of carbs per pound of desired weight.
Maintenance: Consume 2 grams of carbs per pound of desired body weight.
Muscle Gain: Consume 3 grams of carbs per pound of desired body weight.

For fats, the consumption is less than protein and carbs. Because fats contain more than twice the number of calories per gram, the consumption of fats is set as follows:

½ of a gram of fats per pound of desired bodyweight

If this sounds like a lot of work, rest assured that it is not. Once you do this a couple of times, you will remember most of it and not have to figure things out every day with a calculator. Let's do an example:

A person that weighs 200 pounds wants to weigh 190 pounds. Their goal is to lose 10 pounds. The desired body weight is 190 pounds, which we will use in our equations. The macros measurements would look like this:

Protein: 190 grams (x 4) = 760 calories
Carbs: 190 grams (x 4) = 760 calories

Fats: 95 grams (x 9) = 855 calories

Total Calories Daily = 2,375 calories

In this example, the protein and carbohydrate calories are each less than the fat calories allowed in the budget. This is another area in which the individual has the opportunity to customize the program to their own needs. If you are worried about losing weight fast, you can adjust the carbohydrate calories downward. If you are concerned about heart disease, you can adjust the fat intake downward. The idea is to start with the basic equation, as shown above, and then fit the ratio of macro nutrients to meet your specific needs and goals. However, the total calories consumed should stay the same. That means that if you decide to reduce the number of calories you are consuming from fats, you will need to increase the number of calories that you will consume from the protein or carbohydrate groups.

A popular way to get started is to use an equation like 40/40/20. This means that you will devote 40% of your calories to protein, 40% of your calories will come from carbohydrates and 20% of your calories will come from various fats. If you apply this to the above example where the subject needed to consume 2,375 calories each day, the proportions would come out like this:

2,375 calories x 40% = 950 calories from protein
2,375 calories x 40% = 950 calories from carbohydrates
2,375 calories x 20% = 475 calories from fat

By following this formula, and adjusting as you go based on your body's needs, you have the flexibility to accomplish your goals, whatever they may be. It doesn't matter whether you are bulking up, adding lean muscle mass, sliming down, losing sedentary weight or shredding for your next competition, this plan can be customized for you.

Once you have started the process, you can evaluate your body's behavior on a daily and weekly basis, and make adjustments as you go. If you are feeling hungry all the time, increase your protein intake. If you feel tired and lethargic, you may want to consider increasing your fat intake. This process is ongoing, ever-changing and always moving. It is the perfect program for those who want a plan tailored to their individual needs and requirements. As you progress through the steps, you will have flexibility in meals, food choices and meal times as well.

CHAPTER 2

Food Choices

In order to take the next step in constructing your new routine, you will need to decide how many times a day you will plan to have meals. If you are trying to transition from your old habits into a new and improved lifestyle with the least amount of upheaval, you may want to keep it simple at first. Look at what you are already doing and take into account what your current obligations will permit. Are you eating three meals each day? Are you skipping breakfast routinely? Are you forced to eat your final meal at an extremely late hour? Some of these occurences can be altered with a little bit of organization and rescheduling. Unfortunately, some of those obstacles simply cannot be removed easily and must be addressed.

Some exercise experts are proponents of having 5-6 smaller meals each day, which has been known to aid in digestion and the assimilation of the consumed nutrients. Many bodybuilders follow a similar schedule, adjusting their meals around their various workout times. Your schedule may be a bit more limited than that. Perhaps you don't have time to take a lunch, or you have to work through your lunch hour regularly. You may not be able to make it home until late, which makes extensive meal preparation increasingly difficult. If you are a parent, and your child is involved in sports, clubs or any number of after-school activities, you may not arrive back at your kitchen until it is time to send the kids off to bed. All of these situations pose obstacles. If you decide it is worth the work, all of these obstacles can be overcome.

Regardless of how many meals you decide to have, the number of calories that you consume per day must stay the same. The numbers that you came up with back in chapter 1 are your total calories for a single day. Obviously the more meals you have, the smaller they will have to be.

Another area in which you will have an enormous amount of flexibility will be in the foods you choose to eat. The IIFYM diet does not dictate which foods you must consume. The IIFYM diet simply gives you a guideline as to how many calories you need to consume, and from which sources they must be drawn. Your entire day will be filled with choices about which foods to eat and when, and very often you will be tempted to eat empty calories of junk food in place of healthier options. On the IIFYM diet, it doesn't matter if you have a scoop of ice cream or a bran muffin, as long as the item you are consuming fits into your daily caloric intake. This allows the beginner to begin to transition from their old habits to their new behaviors with an ease that other diets do not allow.

If we look back at the example from before, the subject had determined that they needed to stay within 2,375 calories. Let's look at a few different breakdowns that would work within that caloric limit:

You could have 14 cups of mint chocolate chip ice cream. (2,310 calories)
You could eat 12 glazed donuts. (2,304 calories)
You could have 26 cubic inches of fudge. (2,340 calories)
You could devour 95 large marshmallows. (2,375 calories)
You could enjoy 9 nice sized pieces of cheesecake. (2,313 calories.)

Have you ever heard of a diet that would allow this? The idea behind the IIFYM diet is that the food choices are left to the individual, as long as the numbers fit together. This is where we find the origin of the phrase, "If it fits your macros!"

Years ago, there was a diet that allowed you to lose weight by simply eliminating carbs. It didn't matter what you ate, as long as it didn't contain those dreaded carbs. The word spread that this diet actually resulted in rapid weight loss, and common sense went out the window. People started eating double hamburger patties, smothered in mayonnaise and melted cheese, wrapped in strips of whole bacon, dipped in butter. People lost weight, and that diet was immensely popular, until the side effects showed up. You see, eating like that may have caused some of the pounds to come off, but it also caused heart disease, encouraged the growth of cancer cells and raised bad cholesterol to new heights. The idea here is that the individual has the responsibility to say to themselves that just because they *can* eat 95 marshmallows a day, doesn't mean that they *should*.

With great power comes a greater degree of responsibility. This eating plan allows for occassional misteps, cheat days and indulgences. However, these daliances are really only supposed to occur in short spurts and should be balanced by common sense and moderation. The list of junk food above actually works within the framework of the caloric intake limits, but it fails miserably if the individual is committed to sticking to a prescribed course of good health. Looking good is important, but feeling good is essential.

As you move forward on your journey, choosing the foods that work the best in your daily plan will become easier and easier. If you are looking for a good, solid starting point, take a look at what you are doing now. If you prefer chicken over fish, don't try to adopt tilapia and swordfish as dietary staples right off the bat. Stick with the foods you prefer and prepare them in a healthier fashion. If you like broccoli, but you can't stand brussel sprouts, stick with the little green stalks and use them in one of the fantastic recipes that you will find later in this book. You do not need to totally reinvent yourself as you take your first step toward improving your health. You can take it slowly, adapt at your own pace and allow the transition to occur with as little pain and discomfort as possible.

The recipes that are offered for your consideration are as flexible as the eating plan itself. If you like the idea of a cucumber sauce, but not if you have to pour it over a fish filet, then substitute a chicken breast or a patty made from ground turkey. You can adjust the calories, carbs, protein and fats and be on your way. Any of these recipes can be changed in a similar fashion. Keep in mind that it isn't just the main ingredient or the meat product that can be swapped out. Any of the vegetables can be ommitted or added, as long as the nutritional adjutment is made. The side dishes such as angel hair pasta or basmati rice are suggestions based on actual trial and error and are suggested as the best way to have the various foods compliment one another, but they are not written in stone either. Feel free to experiment, substitute or strike out on your own trail. Frankly, that is part of the fun.

CHAPTER 3

Breakfast Recipes

Breakfast is the most important meal of the entire day. I'm sure you have heard that old saying many times before. Have you ever wondered why people believe that to be true? When you rise from your slumber, your metabolism is prepped for the day. Your stomach has had a chance to empty itself out from dinner the night before, and your body has had a chance to filter out a few of the numerous toxins that you come in contact with every day. The first meal of the day is crucial, as this sets the tone for the body to follow until it lays down to sleep once more.

The first meal of the day is absorbed faster and more efficiently than any other meal that will follow it. This means that the nutritional content of that meal will play a major role in providing the body's fuel for the remainder of that day. A meal that contains the proper proportion of macro nutrients that you have determined to be optimal for your body can have long reaching positive results. Unfortunately, a poorly chosen meal consisting of marshmallows and cheesecake will cause long reaching negative effects in much the same manner. These recipes are offered as healthy alternatives to the empty, sugar laden calories that plague us all. They are balanced between protein, carbs and fat and they are relatively low in calories. Once again, please feel free to substitute wherever you wish. All of the recipes provided are designed to serve 1 person. Feel free to double the ingredients for 2 servings, or double it once more in order to serve a family of four.

Santa Fe Spread:

Ingredients:

Half of a ripe avocado
½ tsp lime juice
Half of a whole grain bagel

½ cup strawberries and blueberries
2 slices of turkey bacon

Method:

1. Scoop the ripened avocado from its skin and mash it thoroughly into a thick spread.

2. Add lime juice to taste. Spread over the top of the toasted whole grain bagel.
3. Sprinkle with red pepper flakes to add some zing.
4. Serve with fruit and bacon.

Total calories: 412   Total protein: 12 g   Total carbs: 74 g   Total fats: 20 g

Southwestern Scrambler:

Ingredients:

2 eggs
1 turkey sausage link
1 slice of turkey bacon
2 large tomato slices
1 tbsp shredded Mexican cheese

½ tsp paprika
1 tsp chives
1 tbsp extra virgin olive oil
1 slice whole grain toast

Method:

1. Dice the bacon and sausage and toss in a searing pan with olive oil and chives.
2. Separate the yolks from the egg-whites, whip the whites, and pour over searing bacon and sausage.
3. When cooked, remove from heat, top with tomato slices and sprinkle with paprika and cheese.
4. Cover for 30 seconds to allow cheese to melt.
5. Serve open faced on top of plain toast.

Total calories: 289   Total protein: 14 g   Total carbs: 12 g   Total fat: .07 g

Farmer's Orchard French Toast

Ingredients:

1 slice of whole grain bread
1 egg, whole
2 turkey sausage patties

½ an apple, wedged
1 tbsp almond butter

Method:

1. Crack egg into a bowl and whip.
2. Dip bread into egg mixture, making sure to cover both sides.
3. Coat pan with non-fat cooking spray.

4. Place bread in pan, flip, remove from pan and move to the plate.
5. Rinse pan and coat with melted almond butter.
6. Place sausage patties and apple wedges into sizzling almond butter and cook until prepared.
7. Serve sausage and apples on top of French toast.

Total calories: 360   Total protein: 18 g   Total carbs: 26 g   Total fats: 20 g

Montana Steak & Eggs

Ingredients:

2 eggs, whole
5oz. lean sirloin steak
½ green bell pepper
½ large sweet onion, sliced

½ sweet potato
½ tsp lemon pepper
1 tbsp tamari soy sauce
Extra virgin olive oil, as needed

Method:

1. Toss sirloin steak into a searing pan coated in olive oil and tamari.
2. Let it cook for a few minutes, turning occasionally.
3. Toss in bell pepper and onion, and add olive oil as needed.
4. Plate the steak and add ½ of a cooked sweet potato to the vegetables.
5. Add additional olive oil if needed.
6. Place next to the steak on the plate.
7. Add non-fat cooking spray to the same pan and drop in two eggs.
8. Fry the eggs sunny side up.
9. Add lemon pepper, and serve over the potato and vegetable mixture.

Total calories: 471   Total protein: 42 g   Total carbs: 14 g   Total fats: 25 g

Rodeo Raisin Oat Cake

Ingredients:

½ cup of 1-minute oatmeal
1 tbsp protein powder
¼ cup raisins

2 turkey sausage patties
1 tbsp powdered sugar
1 tbsp yogurt butter

Method:

1. Combine oatmeal, protein powder and yogurt butter in a small mixing bowl.
2. Add water, one tablespoon at a time, until ingredients are mixed together but the batter remains very thick.
3. Add raisins and additional water if needed.
4. Spray a pan with non-stick, non-fat cooking spray.
5. Spread the mixture out in the pan into one large cake, about ½ inch thick.
6. Cook turkey sausage patties in a similar fashion.
7. When finished, place the cake on the plate and the sausage patties on top.
8. Sprinkle with powdered sugar.

Total calories: 391   Total protein: 17 g   Total carbs: 57 g   Total fats: 13 g

These are just a few of the breakfast options available. As you can see, simply using these recipes and substituting different items with similar nutritional properties can change the taste and texture of the entire dish. Following simple variations can give you the variety you crave while still staying within your macros guidelines.

CHAPTER 4

Lunch and Dinner Recipes

L unch and dinner menus are often interchangeable. For that purpose, they are being grouped together in this chapter. As you plan your meal times and your number of meals per day, utilize these recipes to their fullest potential. If you are eating 5 or 6 smaller meals in a day, prepare one of these recipes and split it between two separate meals. If you are opting to have two or three meals per day, you may want to double up on the ingredients to ensure that you are getting enough of the right kind of calories each day.

With breakfast, you have a great deal of flexibility in terms of your selections and caloric intake. When you wake up to start your day, your calorie counter is at zero. Wherever the totals fall for breakfast is irrelevant, as they will be accounted for later in the day. When you get to lunch however, you have to start paying attention to the math. If you are trying to stay within a certain number of calories, you have to start planning ahead when you get to this point in the day. Otherwise, you may be dining on a single Melba toast for dinner.

As the day drags on and we get distracted by events in our everyday lives, the temptation to give up and just eat junk food grows. Plan ahead for the temptation that you know is on its way. Pack healthy, low calorie snacks like carrot sticks, granola bars or almonds into your purse or briefcase. This can head off the temptation before it strikes. Planning, recording and monitoring are the keys to victory in our attempts to change our lives and win the day.

Oriental Braised Beef

Ingredients:

5 oz. lean beef
½ cup water chestnuts
½ cup mushrooms
½ bell pepper

¼ cup brown rice, cooked
Extra virgin olive oil
Teriyaki sauce

Method:

1. Slice the beef into long, thin strips.
2. Place into searing pan with 1 tablespoon of water and 1 tablespoon of olive oil.
3. Flip once, stir, and add the additional ingredients along with 2 tablespoons of teriyaki sauce.
4. This is a fast cooking dish, so it must be stirred constantly.
5. Steam or boil the brown rice according to preference.
6. Spread the beef and vegetables over the rice.

Total Calories: 382   Total Protein: 32 g   Total Carbs: 25 g   Total Fat: 16 g

Tilapia with Cucumber Dressing

Ingredients:

4 oz. boneless tilapia fillet   1 tbsp sour cream
½ cup chopped cucumber, with skin   Dill seasoning
½ cup sliced almonds   5 asparagus spears, large
1 tbsp real mayonnaise

Method:

1. Cut a piece of aluminum foil large enough to wrap around the fillet and seal together with at least two inches of room between the top of the foil and the fish.
2. Place the asparagus spears side by side in the middle of the foil.
3. Rinse the fillet and place it on top of the asparagus.
4. In a separate bowl, combine the chopped cucumber, mayonnaise and sour cream.
5. Add a pinch of dill seasoning.
6. Pour the mixture over the top of the fish, covering it completely.
7. Spread the almonds over the top of the mixture and press into a crust.
8. Bring the ends of the foil together leaving a space above the fish for the steam to collect.
9. Place on a cookie sheet and bake for 8-10 minutes at 375°F.
10. This is an extremely low-carb dish.
11. If your particular needs call for additional carbs, pair this with basmati rice for balanced flavor, then adjust the macro nutrient numbers.

Total calories: 270   Total protein: 25 g   Total carbs: 6 g   Total fat: 16 g

Tuscan Chicken

Ingredients:

4 oz chicken breast, boneless and skinless   10 cherry tomatoes
1 thick slice deli ham   2 tbsp sun dried tomato Italian dressing
1 thick slice Swiss cheese   2 oz. angel hair pasta

Method:

1. Prepare the chicken breast by slicing it laterally.
2. Layer the slice of ham and the slice of Swiss cheese in between the top and bottom pieces of chicken breast.
3. Place the stuffed chicken breast into a small baking dish.
4. Cover with the sun dried tomato dressing.
5. Cover with foil and cook for 20 minutes at 375°F.
6. Prepare the pasta in a separate pot.
7. Place the cooked pasta on a plate, top it with the stuffed chicken and remaining dressing from the baking dish.
8. Garnish with fresh cherry tomatoes.

Total Calories: 484   Total Protein: 38 g   Total Carbs: 53 g   Total Fats: 13 g

Shrimp Creole Salad

Ingredients:

3 oz. cooked shrimp, tail off   ½ cup water chestnuts, sliced
1 cup torn lettuce, green leaf   ½ cup shitake mushrooms
½ avocado, chopped   2 tbsp tiger sauce

Method:

1. Mix all ingredients together in a medium sized mixing bowl.
2. Serve cold.
3. Add a piece of whole grain bread or a roll to the meal to boost carb intake if needed for your personal dietary goals.

Total calories: 280   Total protein: 21 g   Total carbs: 22 g   Total fats: 12 g

Mandarin Chicken Salad

Ingredients:

1 cup shredded lettuce, green leaf
½ cup shredded cabbage
4 oz. boneless, skinless chicken breast, diced
1 tbsp teriyaki sauce
1 tbsp extra virgin olive oil

¼ cup mandarin oranges
1/8 cup bean sprouts
¼ cup sliced water chestnuts
1/8 cup snow peas
2 green onions, diced
2 tbsp low-fat Oriental dressing

Method:

1. Place chicken breast into searing pan coated in olive oil and teriyaki sauce.
2. Slice or dice based on preference.
3. Combine all other ingredients in a medium sized mixing bowl.
4. Stir in cooked chicken and dressing of choice.
5. Serve cold.

Total calories: 249   Total protein: 29 g   Total carbs: 9 g   Total fats: 4 g

Tempting Turkey Burgers

Ingredients:

4 oz. ground turkey breast
½ tbsp Dijon mustard

½ tsp garlic powder
1 green onion, diced

Method:

1. In a small bowl, combine the ground turkey, mustard, garlic powder and green onion.
2. Mix together thoroughly.
3. Form mixture into a patty and grill until done.
4. Serve on a whole grain bun and garnish with lettuce, tomato and pickle.

Total calories: 248   Total protein: 31 g   Total carbs: 21 g   Total fats: 3.5 g

Salsa Swordfish

Ingredients:

6 oz. swordfish steak
½ cup diced tomato
½ cup red onion, chopped
½ tsp lime juice
1 tbsp capers

5 strips bell pepper, (red, orange, yellow or purple.)
1 tbsp balsamic vinaigrette
1 tbsp extra virgin olive oil
1 cup fresh spinach, shredded

Method:

1. Prepare tomato, red onion, lime juice, capers and peppers in a bowl.
2. Crush together into a thick mixture.
3. Place swordfish steak into searing pan with oil and balsamic vinaigrette.
4. Cook swordfish 2-3 minutes per side.
5. Place spinach on plate, top with swordfish, then cover with salsa mixture.

Total calories: 240   Total protein: 38 g   Total carbs: 12 g   Total fats: 7 g

Tasty Tuna Salad

Ingredients:

3 oz. canned tuna in water
½ cup chopped sweet onion
½ cup chopped celery
1 tbsp slivered almonds
1 tbsp light mayonnaise
½ tsp lemon juice
2 large romaine lettuce leaves
1 small tomato, sliced

Method:

1. Combine all ingredients except lettuce and tomato.
2. Mix together thoroughly.
3. Refrigerate before serving.
4. Serve over romaine lettuce leaves and tomato slices.

Total calories: 184   Total protein: 28 g   Total carbs: 4 g   Total fats: 2 g

Sweet Chili Chicken

Ingredients:

4 oz. chicken breast, boneless and skinless

2 tbsp "Chun's" Sweet Chili Sauce

1 cup fresh spinach

1 tbsp extra virgin olive oil

2 tsp garlic powder

1 red potato, chopped

Method:

1. Spray a small baking dish with non-fat, non-stick cooking spray.
2. Layer the bottom of the dish with the spinach.
3. Place the chicken breast in the center of the dish and cover with olive oil, sweet chili sauce and garlic powder.
4. Spread the potatoes around the outside of the dish.
5. Cover with lid or foil and bake for 20 minutes at 375° F.

Total calories: 377   Total protein: 39 g   Total carbs: 57 g   Total fats: 16 g

Sicilian Spaghetti Squash with Meat Sauce

Ingredients:

1 medium spaghetti squash, cooked

1 cup pasta sauce

1 cup ground turkey

½ green bell pepper

¼ sweet onion

1 tbsp extra virgin olive oil

1 tsp garlic powder

Method:

1. Microwave the spaghetti squash for 8 minutes on high to soften it.
2. Remove the squash from the husk and shred.
3. In another pan, brown the turkey, pepper and onion with the olive oil and garlic powder.
4. When ready, toss the squash into the pan and add the sauce.
5. Stir for 2-3 minutes to mix ingredients and warm sauce.
6. Remove from heat and serve.

Total calories: 405   Total protein: 39 g   Total carbs: 41 g   Total fats: 27 g

Portobello Pizza

Ingredients:

1 large Portobello mushroom cap

¼ cup marinara sauce

¼ cup green pepper, chopped

¼ cup shredded mozzarella cheese, part-skim, low-fat

Method:

1. Heat the oven to 375° F.
2. Place the flattened mushroom cap on a cookie sheet or baking stone.
3. Cover with sauce, add toppings and cheese.
4. Bake for 10 minutes or until the cheese is golden.

Total calories: 155   Total protein: 12 g   Total carbs: 14 g   Total fats:7 g

Honey Dijon Pork Medallion

Ingredients:

4 oz. pork loin

1 tsp lemon pepper

1 tbsp yogurt butter

2 tbsp lemon juice

1 tbsp Worcestershire sauce

1 tbsp honey

1 tsp Dijon mustard

1 tbsp chopped fresh parsley

½ cup brown rice

Method:

1. Prepare rice as needed, according to the type and brand.
2. Place pork loin in small baking dish.
3. In a small bowl, mix all other ingredients.
4. Pour mixture over pork loin and bake at 400° F for 10 minutes.
5. Serve cooked pork and sauce from baking dish over rice.

Total calories: 330   Total protein: 24 g   Total carbs: 24 g   Total fats: 17 g

Turkey Tortilla Roll Up

Ingredients:

1 whole wheat tortilla

5 slices of thinly sliced turkey breast

1 cup leafy romaine lettuce

1 tsp Dijon mustard

4 slices of cucumber, skin on

1/3 cup green bell pepper, diced

Method:

1. Layer the turkey into the center of the heated tortilla.
2. Layer additional ingredients into the tortilla evenly.
3. Roll tortilla tightly and enjoy.
4. This is a great snack or meal for individuals with extremely busy schedules.

Total calories: 218   Total protein: 15 g   Total carbs: 30 g   Total fats: 3 g

Hawaiian Chicken Medley

Ingredients:

4 oz. chicken breast, boneless, skinless

¼ cup pineapple juice

½ cup brown rice, cooked

1 cup frozen mixed vegetables

Method:

1. Prepare the vegetables in a microwave safe dish with a cup of water.
2. Heat in the microwave for 5-6 minutes or until hot.
3. Prepare the brown rice as directed by the brand and specific serving instructions.
4. In a large frying pan, cook the chicken breast in the pineapple juice and some water as needed, until thoroughly cooked through.
5. Without draining the pineapple juice from the pan, strain the vegetables and add them to the pan.
6. Add the cooked rice.
7. Mix together and serve as a single dish.

Total calories: 353   Total protein: 32 g   Total carbs: 46 g   Total fats: 6 g

Grilled Citrus Salmon

Ingredients:

4 oz. wild salmon fillet
1 tbsp lemon juice
1 tbsp orange juice
1 tbsp lime juice

1 tsp red pepper flakes
1 tsp black pepper
2 green onions
1 cup arugula, chopped

Method:

1. Spray the bottom and sides of a small baking dish with non-fat, non-stick cooking spray.
2. Place the green onions in the shape of an "X" in the dish.
3. Place the salmon fillet on top of the onion.
4. In a separate small bowl combine the lemon, orange and lime juices.
5. Pour over the top of the salmon.
6. Cover with spices.
7. Pack arugula on top of the salmon to keep the juices and spices from running off.
8. Cover and bake at 375°F for 10 minutes.

Total calories: 210   Total protein: 28 g   Total carbs: 8 g   Total fats: 4 g

CHAPTER 5

The Workout, Stage 1

Stage 1: The Beginner

The recommended workouts for this exercise plan are low impact but highly effective. Based on your age and level of activity, there are three different workout plans that are recommended. They focus on strengthening your joints, tendons and ligaments and reducing your bodyweight. There are additional programs that can be found online for bulking up or adding lean muscle mass. For the purposes of this book, the focus will be on weight loss and improved motion range. As with any workout plan, you may want to consult your physician before adopting a new lifestyle.

This stage is recommended for older individuals who suffer from injuries or ailments that impede their movement. People with bad knees, chronic back pain, rotator cuff injuries, plantar fasciitis, arthritis or any similar type of painful condition should start here. This program is also recommended for individuals of any age that have been seriously sedentary for a period of more than 2 years, or those that are battling a severe weight problem. This program is designed to get you off the couch, out of the house and back in motion. The focus is on stretching and getting the blood flowing in and out of those unused muscles. The idea is to bring back some vitality and movement in areas that have become dormant. The more you can do, the better you feel. By progressing through this basic beginner program, you will be increasing your range of motion, improving your circulation and blood flow and producing and releasing endorphins into your system that simply make you feel better.

The basic exercise for this plan is walking. You can walk around your block, through your neighborhood or anywhere that you feel safe and secure. If you need to, you can drive to a location where you feel comfortable enough to get out and walk. You will start off with three days each week, walking for at least 30 minutes. This will be the foundation for your workout plan until you are ready to advance to the next stage. While you are walking, here are a few guidelines to remember:

Stand up straight, or as straight as you can. This helps to improve posture and strengthens the abdominal and lower back muscles that make up your core.

Move along at a brisk pace that makes you push and sweat, but not so fast that you are out of breath. If you can't have a phone conversation while you are walking, slow down.

Keep a journal of when you start, when you finish and how you felt. Try to go a little longer every time until you reach 60 minutes of walking.

In addition to walking, you need to start stretching. Basic stretches for your major muscle groups should be done daily, regardless of whether or not you are planning a workout that day. When you stretch, you are forcing your muscles to expand and contract in a way that is different from their normal daily routine. As you do the stretching, tiny capillaries come apart and there is some breaking down of muscle tissue.

This is what you are looking for. This action causes blood to course through those muscles in an increased capacity. More blood in the muscle means more oxygen is being transported to that muscle. Oxygen, along with nutrients found in the blood, are essential for the growth and recovery of the muscle groups you are targeting. Basic stretches will bring about plenty of activity in this area. A list of those stretches has been compiled below.

Toe Touches: Stand with your feet together, knees slightly bent and shoulders back. Lean forward slowly and try to touch your toes. If you can't quite make it that's perfectly fine. Be sure not to bounce when you are in the downward position. Hold your stretch for a count of ten and then slowly rise back up to a standing position. Once you are back in the starting position, reach your hands straight back up over your head as if you were trying to touch the sky. Reach up with your hands and flex your fingers as you open and close them. Do this for a count of ten and return to the standing position with your hands at your sides. That is 1 repetition. You need to do 5 of these.

Swimmer Stretch: Stand straight, feet shoulder width apart, arms hanging loosely at your sides. Raise your arms until they are directly in front of you, hands open with palms facing each other. Gently push your palms together for a count of ten. Relax, then with your arms extended move your arms behind you as if you are trying to touch them together behind your back. Look upward and lean your head back slightly to accentuate this stretch. Hold for a count of ten. That is 1 repetition. You need to do 5 of these.

Calves and Feet: Face the nearest wall and lean against it with your palms flat and your fingers pointing upward. Relax your body and step backward, placing your foot on the ground gently. This will cause a massive stretching of the muscles in the bottom of your foot, ankle, heel and calf muscles. Hold for a ten count. Gently and slowly pick that foot up and step backward with the other foot, lightly pressing against the wall for stability and resistance. Repeat the procedure. Hold both stretches for a count of 10.

Once you have done that for both feet, you will have accomplished 1 repetition. You need to do 5 of these.

Performing these stretches at least three times each week, preferably before you go for your walk, will exponentially increase the oxygen levels in your blood stream, and it will decrease the discomfort you will feel both during the walk and afterward. As you progress, you will want to increase the amount of time you spend walking until you get to 60 minutes for each session. Once you are successfully walking for 60 minutes, 3 times each week, add a fourth session. Continue this until you feel that you are ready for Stage 2.

CHAPTER 6

The Workout, Stage 2

Stage 2: The Weekend Warrior

S tage two is for the moderate athlete, the weekend warrior, the person who makes the occasional yoga class but doesn't know the instructor's name, etc. This stage is designed to take a person who is *somewhat* active and help them to become *very* active. This program will help you reach the next level in your training so that you can advance into a state of beginning competition in some activity. People who are at this stage understand some of the basic terminology, such as "sets" and "reps." You will need a small amount of equipment for this stage, such as exercise bands, weights, proper cross training or running shoes and similar items.

This program comes with a word of caution however, for anyone who believes that they are at this level. Too often people jump into a workout plan assuming that they can handle the level of activity called for even though they have not performed that activity, at that level in many years. Take an honest accounting of your body. Look for the aches and pains that are warning signs of serious injuries waiting to happen. Examine yourself for sharp discomfort when you walk, run or stretch. If you have any issues that may be a cause for concern, simply start with Stage 1. You do not need to stay at that stage for any prescribed period of time. You can simply start there, get used to your body and how it works and take a slightly slower approach to your progression. Allow your body to catch up with your motivation and the two shall meet later on down the road under much more pleasant circumstances.

Stage 2 is a resistance based approach that revolves around a 4-day training schedule. You can adjust the planned sessions to be performed on different days, but it is important to leave the weekends alone for now. If you are reading this book, the chances are extremely good that you are very busy with your job, your family or your daily activities. Trying to utilize all of your available time to craft a new workout program when you are already pressed for time, is a recipe for defeat. In the interest of continuity, the following program is based on 4 workouts that take place on the assigned days, as listed below:

MONDAY / THURSDAY:

Stretch.

20 minutes of aerobic activity designed to raise the heart rate, such as running, walking, using the elliptical machine, riding a bike, etc.

Resistance training. Weights or Exercise bands. Targeting major muscle groups in the upper body. Individual exercises listed later. Optimal duration: 40 minutes.

TUESDAY / FRIDAY:

Stretch.

20 minutes of aerobic activity designed to raise the heart rate, such as running, walking, using the elliptical machine, riding a bike, etc.

Resistance training. Weights or Exercise bands. Targeting major muscle groups in the lower body. Individual exercises listed later. Optimal duration: 40 minutes.

This workout schedule allows for 2 days of solid exercise, both high energy and low impact, without placing the individual in danger of overtraining or injury. The first two days are followed by a Wednesday that is an "off" day, allowing the body time to rest and recuperate. Then we hit it again on Thursday and Friday, allowing for Saturday and Sunday to be days of rest and recovery. Do what you need to do to work around your personal schedules and obligations, but do your best to leave Saturday and Sunday out of the mix.

During the resistance portion of the workout, these exercises will provide a single, solid, reliable movement for each of the main muscle groups, allowing you to build a strong foundation. Once you have performed these specific exercises, and you have developed a feel for the way they impact the muscle group they are targeting, you can substitute other exercises in their place as you progress.

Upper Body Exercises:

CHEST: Bench Press. Lie on a workout bench, holding your weights or resistance bands at the sides of your chest and push upward, away from your chest. At full extension, your arms should be holding the weights directly above your chest, below your chin and above your midsection. If you do not have weights or a weight bench, you can lie on the floor with a resistance band secured underneath you, running directly across your shoulder blades. Push upward against the resistance. Your goal is to be able to complete 3 sets of 10 reps. At that point, increase the weight or resistance and continue.

BACK: One Armed Rows. Stand above your workout bench, with your right knee and right hand supporting your weight across the bench. You should be facing the floor at this point. Reach down and pick up your weight, pulling it to your side. Your elbow will be raised above your torso. Lower the weight back down, feeling the stretch in the muscles along the side of your back. That is 1 repetition. Your goal is to complete 3 sets of 10 reps without fail.

BICEPS: One Arm Curls. Hold the dumbbell loosely at your side. Rotate your hand so your palm is facing front. Lift the dumbbell upward in an arcing motion until it is ¾ of the way to your shoulder. Hold briefly, then return it to its starting position. Your goal is to complete 3 sets of 12-15 repetitions.

TRICEPS: Extensions. Hold the dumbbell in both hands, behind your head, touching the back of your neck. Do your best to keep your elbows pointing towards the front, as opposed to flaring out. Raise the dumbbell with both hands until your arms are fully extended. Hold, then lower the dumbbell to its starting position behind your head. Your goal is to accomplish 3 sets of 12-15 repetitions each.

SHOULDERS: Military Press. Hold two dumbbells, one in each hand, positioned above your shoulders. Your hands will be pointing upward and your palms will face forward. The dumbbells will be raised and lowered in a straight plane, from the top of the chest until the arms are fully extended. Your goal is to perform and complete 3 sets of 10 repetitions without fail.

Lower Body Exercises:

THIGHS: Squats. The most basic lower body exercise in the world is the squat. This can be performed with or without weights, and can be done with a full or a partial knee bend. Stand straight with your feet slightly wider than shoulder width apart. Bend your knees and lower your body towards the ground. Your upper body will move forward, to compensate for your rear end moving backward. Keep your back straight and your head and eyes up throughout the movement to avoid injury. Lower your body as low as you can without falling, then raise yourself back up to a standing position. That is considered 1 repetition. Your goal is to complete 5 sets of 10 repetitions.

CALVES: Calf Raise. This is another movement that you can do with or without weights based on your muscular development. Stand flat with your legs shoulder width apart. If you are using weights for added resistance, hold them at your sides with your arms outstretched. While keeping your body straight and firm, shift your weight forward and raise yourself upward using just your calves and ankles. At the top of the movement, you will be standing up on your tip-toes. Hold for a 5 count, then lower yourself back down to the standing position. Your goal is to perform 5 sets of 12-15 repetitions.

LOWER BACK: Hyperextensions. This exercise blends in perfectly with the rest of your leg workout. The lower back muscles are used to stabilize the body in virtually every lower body movement. Stand straight with your feet shoulder width apart and your knees bent slightly. With your hands on your hips, bend at the waist, keeping your head and eyes up. Lower your upper body until it forms a 90° angle with your legs. Hold for a count of 5 and slowly raise your torso into an upright position. Your goal is to perform 5 sets of 15-20 repetitions.

ABDOMINALS: Crunches. This exercise strengthens the upper abdominal muscles without putting strain on your lower back. Lie on the floor with your feet raised. You can place them on a couch or a chair, the stairway in your house or whatever will allow your feet to be above your rear end. Slowly raise your shoulders up off of the floor and exhale. You want to raise your shoulders until they are at a 45° angle with the floor. Hold that position for a count of 5 then lower your shoulders back to the floor. Immediately perform the movement again. Your goal is to perform 5 sets of 15-20 repetitions.

ABDOMINALS: Leg Lifts. This exercise strengthens the lower abdominals which press against the muscles of the lower back in maintaining a healthy core. Lie on the floor with your hands tucked underneath the outside edges of your rear end. Slowly lift your feet until your feet and legs are off of the floor and hold them at a height of about 6 inches. Hold for a count of 5, then lower them back down. Immediately repeat the movement. Your goal is to complete 5 sets of 15-20 repetitions.

This intermediate program will help most individuals to take the next step in their training evolution. This is not for beginners or novices. This program, when followed faithfully, will bring about positive results that will be noticeable within the first 6-8 weeks. Stay on this program until you are ready for the final stage.

CHAPTER 7

The Workout, Stage 3

Stage 3: Advanced

In Stage #3, the Advanced Stage, you have risen above the previous two levels of transition and may be ready for a competition of some kind, a tournament or a new regimen that provides some extreme challenges. Whether you are preparing for a marathon, a triathlon, or a weight lifting event, this stage is where you take your level of commitment to an entirely new level. At this point, the exercises that you are doing have advanced beyond the basic bench press, and you are undoubtedly already experimenting with various angles of fly and cable movements. People who have reached this pinnacle are utilizing the IIFYM diet for all that it is worth. They are counting their calories to the decimal point and choosing the healthiest alternatives available. Individuals who reach this level are looking for ways to change their already intense workouts and are trying to break through their current plateaus and make additional gains.

It is time now to tailor your weight resistance program to your particular needs. Unlike the weekend warrior from the last stage, you don't need a one-size-fits-all regiment. As you set your goals, the program that you need will become evident.

These programs can be divided into two basic categories; endurance training and strength training. If you are considering a marathon for instance, that activity requires that your body be able to perform at a high level over a great distance, for a long time. This qualifies as an endurance event, and your training should be formulated to match. You will need to change the number of repetitions that you do. You should be performing exercises using 25 to 35 reps. This will cause your muscles to adapt to longer workouts, and teach them how to handle stress that is administered over a longer time period. As you reach the 10th mile of your marathon, you need your muscles to be on the same track physically that you are mentally.

You will also change some of the exercises that you are doing to fit the program that you are trying to build. A marathon runner wants strong arms of course, but not arms that are growing larger and heavier with each workout. This will cause you limit your arm workouts to one or two movements, and use lighter weights for an extended period of time. Your leg workouts will increase however, as you build those muscles for endurance racing. However, you will still not be looking to increase the overall size and weight of your legs, as that would hinder your running times as opposed to helping them.

For strength training, you will build your program to opposing goals from the endurance regiment that we just described. If you are competing in a weight lifting or bodybuilding competition, or competing in a physical, power sport such as football or rugby, then you will need to build larger, stronger muscles that can perform the needed tasks and protect your body from injury. Shorter repetitions with heavier weights will be the course of the day, and you will be working in the 6-8 rep range as you pack on muscle and strengthen your frame. You will concentrate on basic movements like those described in the last chapter, but you will use the heaviest weights possible and do them in a sequence that maximizes your explosive growth. These workouts are shorter, but they can be even more intense because of the rapid fire muscle building that is taking place as you push yourself to move heavier weights with each session.

As far as individual exercises, people who achieve this level of fitness are already flush with magazines, websites and courses on how to perform movements differently and how to add muscle, drop weight or increase performance. Yet there are a few nuances about breaking out of your training rut that should be mentioned here.

Keep Your Muscles Guessing: Too often we find ourselves doing the same exercises over and over, in the same order, with the same weights and the same number of reps. In order to spur your body into another dimension of improvement, you must occasionally change things up. Try reversing the order of your exercises. Try using heavier weights for a lower number of repetitions or using lighter weights for a higher number of repetitions than usual. Try doing a movement with a different hand grip, or try changing the speed of your movements. Any of these things can make your body wake up and realize that something new is going on.

Alter Your Meal Plan: Try using leaner portions of the meats that you have come to enjoy and rely on. Use different sauces in your preparations. Use a new spice that you haven't tried before, or use an alternative method of cooking that you aren't used to. All of these things can wake up your taste buds and challenge your body to assimilate something different for a change.

Take a Break: Yes, you read that right. After you have waged war on mediocrity for months and months, your body will begin to get used to the fight. Take a break from your training schedule for one week. Do some different activities. Take a vacation. Allow yourself to take some time to sit on the back porch with a glass of fine wine and take a deep breath. Sometimes this recovery will give you a gigantic burst when you return to your training. Sometimes…less is more.

These are just a few of the methods that professional athletes and modern day bodybuilders are using to keep their workouts fresh. By mixing things up, changing your routines or even just giving your body a rest you can stay sharp and keep improving. But how do you know when you have reached one of these sticking points? How do you know when your body has gone from adapting to change to a state of overtraining? Here are a few warning signs to watch out for:

You have not increased the weight you are working with in over a month.

You have trouble concentrating at work, at home, or during your workout.

You are doing the same workout that you have always done, but your appearance is changing negatively.

Your muscles are no longer sore after your workouts, you just feel tired.

Your overall energy level is starting to wither.

By keeping a constant vigil on these issues, you will be able to stop yourself from hitting this barrier and losing precious time. There are many other signs as well, and you will have to learn to listen to your body and identify them as you continue down the path you have chosen.

Conclusion

The IIFYM diet plan is a flexible and simple way to give yourself a chance at a new life. You will no longer have to guess about what foods to eat or in what quantities. You will no longer have to wonder about what workout to do or when to do it. The plan allows you to eat virtually anything you want, as long as you eat it in the right amounts. You are primed for success as you set out on this new chapter in your life. Yet, for all of this planning and preparation there is still something missing. There is still one more ingredient that must be added to this mix before you will truly achieve your goals. That thing that is missing is belief.

The IIFYM diet has been carefully researched and constructed so that you can follow it easily. Without your belief however, it will simply remain as words on a page, and not a pathway to success. As you take your first steps toward a new life, you must take that leap of faith and commit yourself to following this plan. The IIFYM diet can be perfectly planned, but without your execution that plan will fail. The exercises can be scheduled, but without your willpower to get up off the couch and perform the movements, they won't produce results.

Ask yourself why you purchased this book. The odds are that you were searching for something new and different. You may have been searching for a healthier lifestyle. Perhaps you were searching for a way to finally lose those extra pounds that you have been carrying around. You may have been looking for a sensible way to improve your self-image without buying a bunch of supplements or diet pills. Whatever the reason, you are in possession of this book now. Your life has changed already, before you even counted a calorie or stretched a single muscle.

Your life has changed, because you now have the power. You now possess the power to change your life. You can wait for a while and think about it, or you can start today. You can make a decision, make a commitment, make a choice…and start today. Only you can make this happen. Only you can pick up this book, and begin to build yourself a better tomorrow. What have you got to lose?

The IIFYM diet gives you all of the tools you need to start constructing a better future. Take advantage of this opportunity. Decide to start right now. When you begin to prepare your next meal, don't change a thing. Cook what you usually cook, the way you usually cook it. However, this time, when you are preparing the food, pay attention to how that particular food fits into your macros numbers. How many calories are in that particular dish? How much protein, carbohydrates or fat are in those ingredients? If you were on the macros diet right now, how would this meal affect you and your plan for the rest of the day?

As you look at your habits through slightly different glasses, you may just start to see some things differently. Usually, people who undertake this exercise are shocked to find out that their current menu is fairly compatible with their new vision. There may be some small tweaks here or there, but the food they are eating fits into the plan pretty well. This plan is flexible for a reason; it is designed to help you achieve success. If you bring the will, this book will show you the way.

Finally, if you enjoyed this book, then I'd like to ask you for a favor, would you be kind enough to leave a review for this book on Amazon? It'd be greatly appreciated!

Be sure to check out our website at www.thetotalevolution.com for more information.

Thank you!

Our Other Books

Below you'll find some of our other books that are popular on Amazon.com and the international sites.

Master Cleanse: How To Do A Natural Detox The Right Way And Lose Weight Fast

Mayo Clinic Diet: A Proven Diet Plan For Lifelong Weight Loss

Glycemic Index Diet: A Proven Diet Plan For Weight Loss and Healthy Eating With No Calorie Counting

Clean Eating Diet: A 10 Day Diet Plan To Eat Clean, Lose Weight And Supercharge Your Body

Wheat Belly: The Anti-Diet - A Guide To Gluten Free Eating And A Slimmer Belly

The Dukan Diet: A High Protein Diet Plan To Lose Weight And Keep It Off For Life

Mediterranean Diet: 101 Ultimate Mediterranean Diet Recipes To Fast Track Your Weight Loss & Help Prevent Disease

Acid Reflux Diet: A Beginner's Guide To Natural Cures And Recipes For Acid Reflux, GERD And Heartburn

Hypothyroidism Diet: Natural Remedies & Foods To Boost Your Energy & Jump Start Your Weight Loss

It Starts With Food: A 30 Day Diet Plan To Reset Your Body, Lose Weight And Become A Healthier You

www.ingramcontent.com/pod-product-compliance
Lightning Source LLC
Chambersburg PA
CBHW030547290526
45786CB00004B/1906